PCOS RECIPES COOKBOOK FOR BEGINNERS

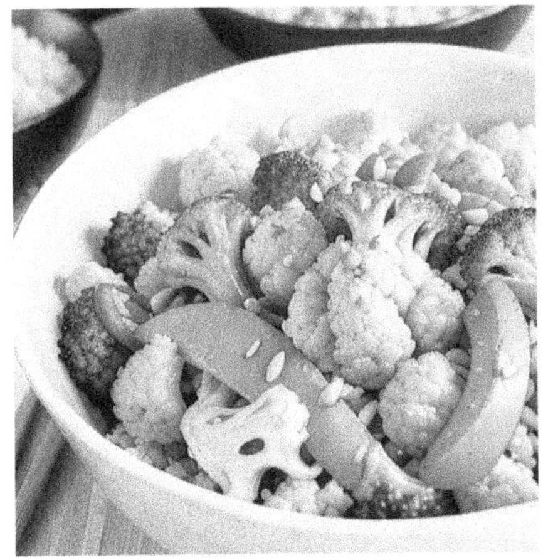

The Ultimate Quick and Easy Delicious Diet

JESSICA MURRAY

Dear Reader,

Thank you for the purchase. I hope you enjoy and love it, would you consider dropping an honest feedback/review, I will appreciate that and you can contact me using JessicaMurrayDietHelp@gmail.com if you have any questions, I will gladly respond

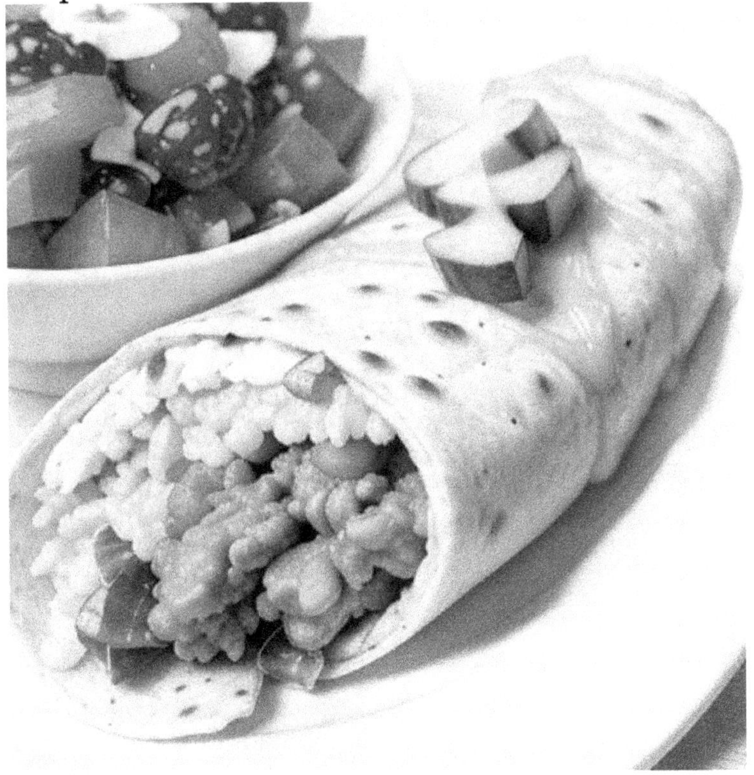

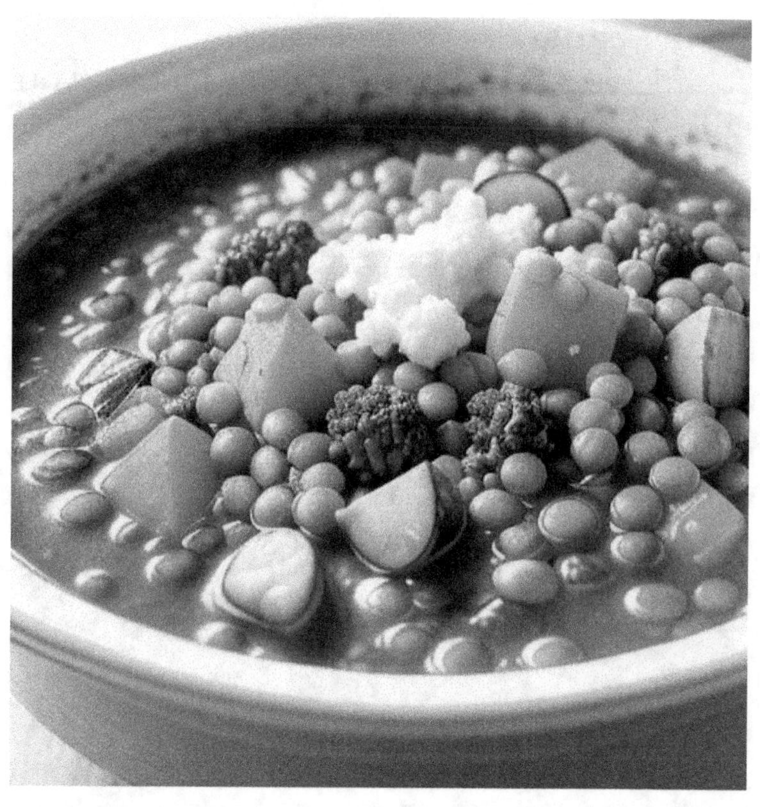

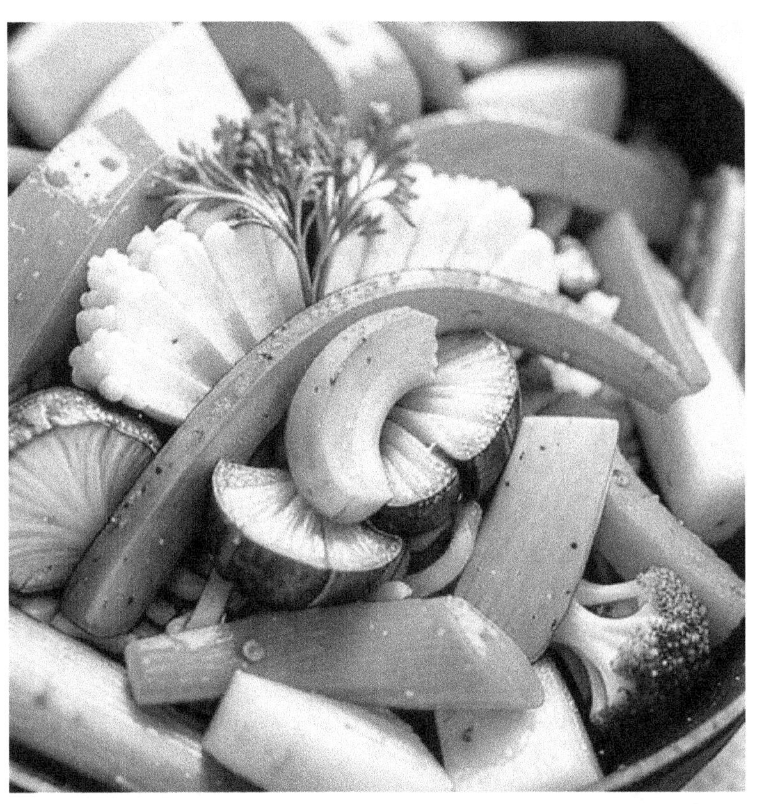

Table of Contents

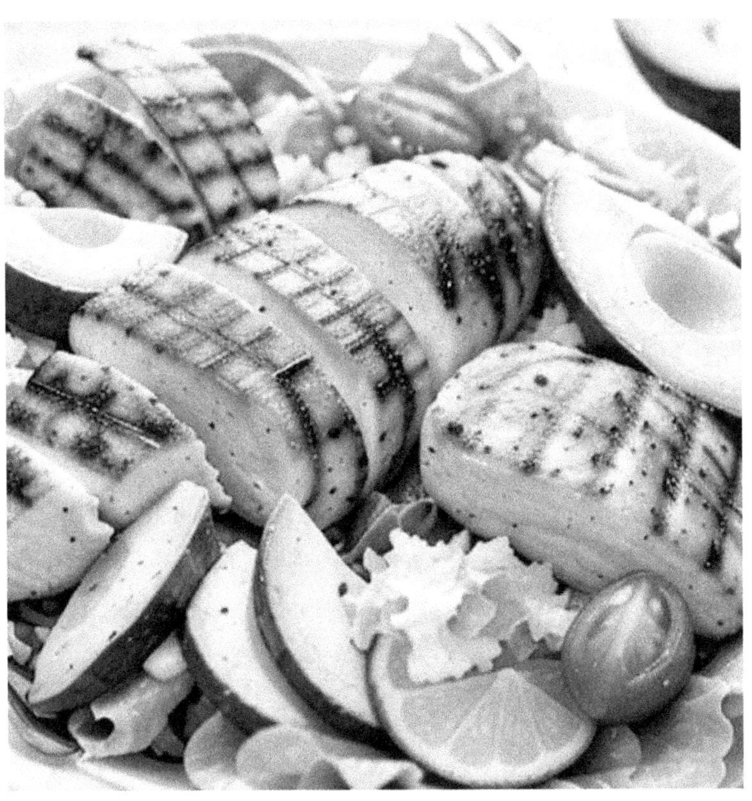

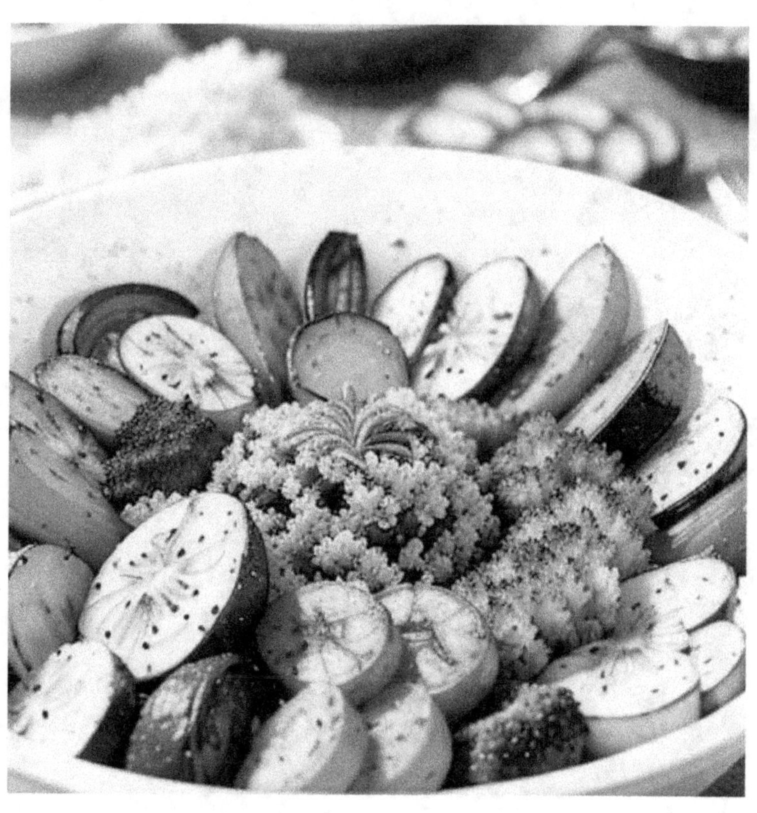

INTRODUCTION TO PCOS

Maya had always liked food, but because of her illness, it was difficult for her to eat without thinking about how it would affect her health. She made the decision to educate herself on PCOS-friendly foods and cooking methods after becoming frustrated by the lack of possibilities. Maya began experimenting in her kitchen with the aid of online resources and a helpful community.

Even though she encountered obstacles along the way, such as burned dishes and failed attempts, Maya persisted. She learned about the strength of whole foods including lean proteins, veggies high in fibre, and complex carbohydrates. She gradually built up a collection of delectable, wholesome meals that were easy on her body.

Maya's perseverance not only improved her health but also served as an example for others.

Maya's tale eventually turned into an example of the impact one person's perseverance may have. By mastering the skill of cooking, she not only overcame the difficulties posed by PCOS but also inspired a community to adopt better lifestyles. Maya's story proved that anyone could find their way to wellness one recipe at a time with a little bit of willpower and a lot of encouragement.

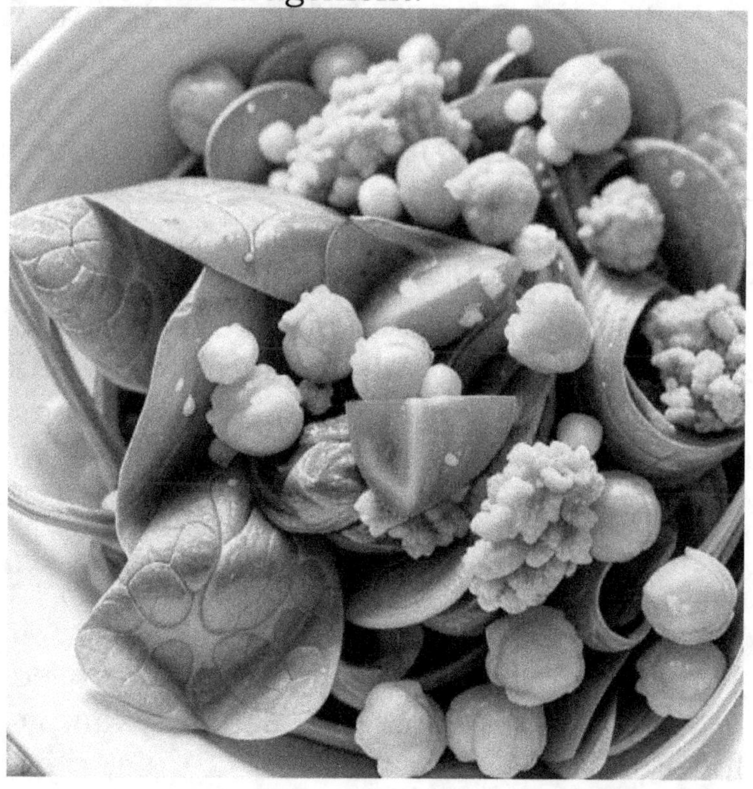

CHAPTER 1

What exactly is PCOS?

A prevalent hormonal condition that mostly affects persons with ovaries during their reproductive years is polycystic ovary syndrome (PCOS).

Combinations of symptoms linked to hormone abnormalities define PCOS. Genetics and insulin resistance are thought to be contributing factors even if the exact cause is not entirely understood. A few of the main characteristics of PCOS include:

1. Unusually long menstrual cycles Due to unpredictable ovulation, people with PCOS may have irregular or non-existent menstrual cycles.

2. Ovarian cysts: Despite the name, not all people with PCOS have ovarian cysts. Multiple tiny follicles on the ovaries are referred to as "polycystic" growths.

Effect On Health

First, fertility Ovulation irregularities can make it difficult to get pregnant. However, many PCOS sufferers can have healthy pregnancies with the right care.

2. Metabolic Results: Due to the prevalence of insulin resistance associated with PCOS, the body may produce more insulin than usual. This raises the risk of type 2 diabetes and weight gain, respectively.

3. Weight Gain Having PCOS makes it difficult for many people to control their weight because of insulin resistance and hormonal imbalances. The signs of PCOS might be made worse by being overweight.

4. Cardiovascular Health: Particularly in overweight individuals, PCOS is linked to a higher risk of heart disease, high blood pressure, and unhealthy cholesterol levels.

5. Mental Wellness: Emotional health may be impacted by PCOS-related hormonal and physical changes. In those with PCOS, depression, anxiety, and low self-esteem are more prevalent.

Diagnoses and Treatment Include

Examining symptoms, medical history, and doing testing to rule out other illnesses are all necessary steps in the PCOS diagnosis process. Treatment plans are individualized to meet each patient's needs and may consist of:

1. Changes to Your Lifestyle Weight management and improved insulin sensitivity can be achieved with regular exercise and a well-balanced diet.

2. Medications Hormonal birth control can control symptoms including acne and excessive hair growth as well as menstrual cycles. To increase insulin sensitivity, a doctor may give the diabetes drug metformin.

3. Fertility Treatments: Ovulation-inducing drugs and assisted reproductive technologies can be helpful for those who are attempting to get pregnant.

4. Mental health support: Dealing with the emotional effects of PCOS through therapy or counselling helps enhance general wellbeing.

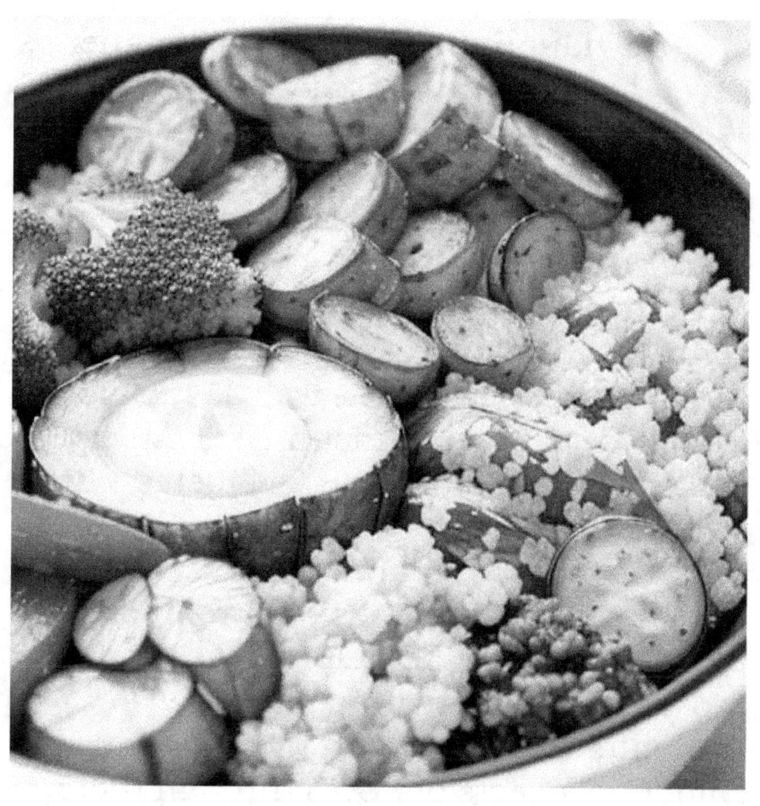

CHAPTER 2

BREAKFAST RECIPES

Berry and Greek Yogurt Parfait

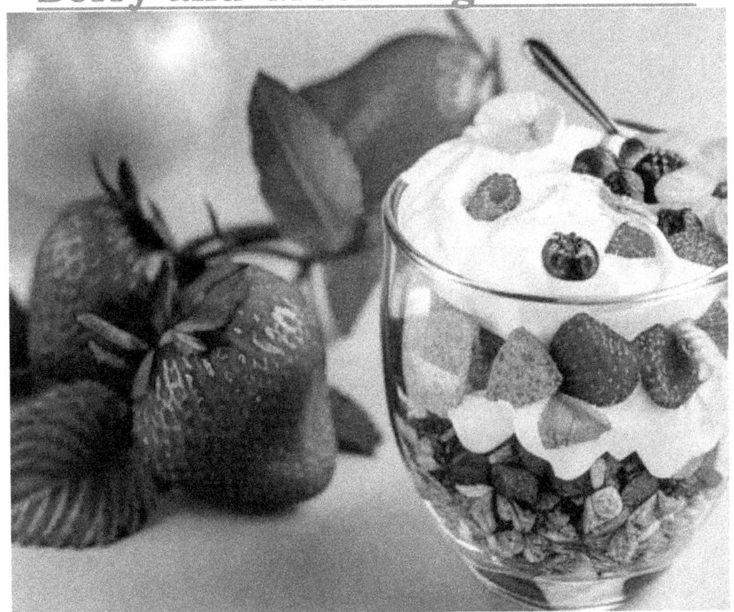

INGREDIENTS

- 1 cup of berries, either fresh or frozen
- One cup of Greek yogurt, plain
- 2 teaspoons of optional honey

INSTRUCTION

- Combine the berries and honey in a medium bowl.
- Spread a layer of Greek yogurt in the bottom of a glass dish.

- Top the yogurt with a layer of the berries and honey mixture.
- Present cold.

Veggie-Packed Breakfast Burritos

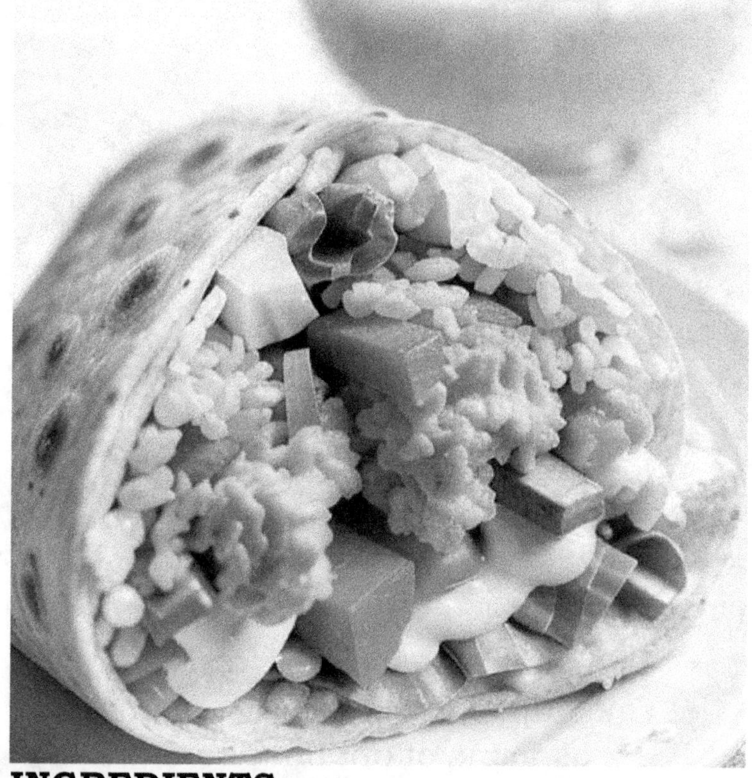

INGREDIENTS

- 2 tablespoons olive oil
- 8 eggs
- 1 chopped red bell pepper
- One cup of chopped mushrooms
- 1/2 cup of onion, diced

- A quarter-teaspoon of smoked paprika
- To taste, salt and pepper
- 2 cups of cheddar cheese, shredded
- 8 soft tortillas in the shape of burritos

INSTRUCTION

- In a large skillet placed over heat of medium-high intensity, the olive oil was heated.
- Add the bell pepper, mushrooms, and onion and simmer, stirring frequently, for about 5 minutes, or until the veggies are tender.
- Add the eggs to the skillet and stir-fry them until they are fully done.
- Salt, pepper, and smoked paprika are used to season the eggs.
- Scoop a portion of the egg mixture onto a tortilla and place it on a dish. grate some cheese on top.
- Wrap the left and right sides of the tortilla around the filling after folding the bottom over.
- Carry out step 7 using the remaining tortillas and filling.

Quinoa Breakfast Bowl

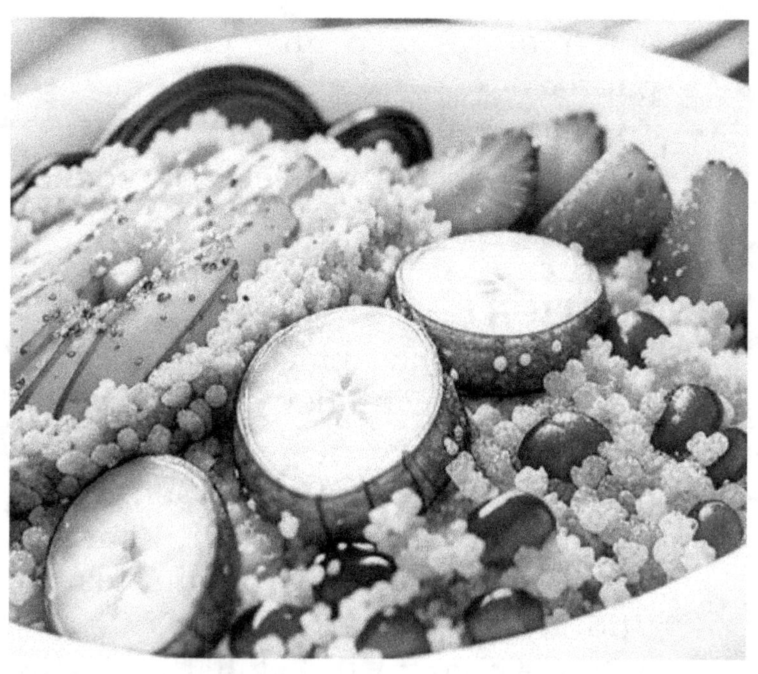

INGREDIENTS

- 1 cup cooked quinoa
- 2 eggs
- 2 tablespoons olive oil
- 1/2 cup of bell peppers, diced
- 1/2 cup of onion, diced
- 2 minced garlic cloves
- A quarter-teaspoon of smoked paprika
- To taste, salt and pepper
- 1/4 cup of feta cheese crumbles

INSTRUCTION

- In a medium skillet over medium-high heat, warm the olive oil.
- Include the bell pepper, onion, and garlic and simmer for 5 minutes, or until the vegetables are tender.
- Include the eggs in the skillet and fry them until they are fully done.
- Salt, pepper, and smoked paprika are used to season the eggs.
- Distribute the quinoa into two bowls, then top each with feta cheese crumbles and half of the egg mixture.
- Present hot.

Vegetable Omelette

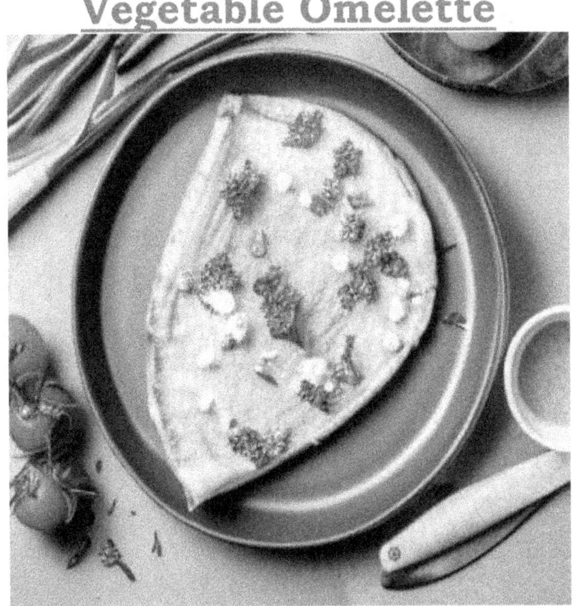

INGREDIENTS

- 2 tablespoons olive oil
- 1/2 cup of bell pepper, chopped
- 1/4 cup finely minced onion
- A cup and a half of chopped mushrooms
- 2 minced garlic cloves
- 4 eggs
- 1/4 cup of finely chopped cheese
- To taste, salt and pepper

INSTRUCTION

- In a medium skillet over medium-high heat, warm the olive oil.
- Add the bell pepper, onion, mushrooms, and garlic and simmer, stirring frequently, for about 5 minutes, or until the veggies are tender.
- Combine the eggs in a medium bowl and season with salt and pepper.
- After adding the egg mixture to the skillet, cook the eggs while stirring occasionally until they are set.
- Cheese-sprinkle the omelette, then fold it in half.
- Present hot.

Spinach and Mushroom Breakfast Wrap

Ingredients:

- 2 tablespoons olive oil
- One cup of chopped mushrooms
- One-fourth teaspoon of dried oregano
- 2 minced garlic cloves
- Two cups baby spinach
- 4 eggs
- four whole wheat tortillas
- 1/4 cup of finely chopped cheese
- To taste, salt and pepper

Instructions:

- In a medium skillet over medium-high heat, warm the olive oil.
- Include the oregano and mushrooms, and simmer for 5 minutes or until the mushrooms are browned.
- Include the garlic and heat for approximately a minute, or until fragrant.
- Include the spinach and simmer for one minute, or until wilted.
- Combine the eggs in a small bowl and season with salt and pepper.

- Using a skillet, add the egg mixture, and cook while stirring occasionally until the eggs are set.
- Distribute the egg mixture among the tortillas that are still warm and top with cheese.
- Roll the tortillas up, then warmly serve.

CHAPTER 3

Wholesome Lunches
Avocado with Grilled Chicken Salad

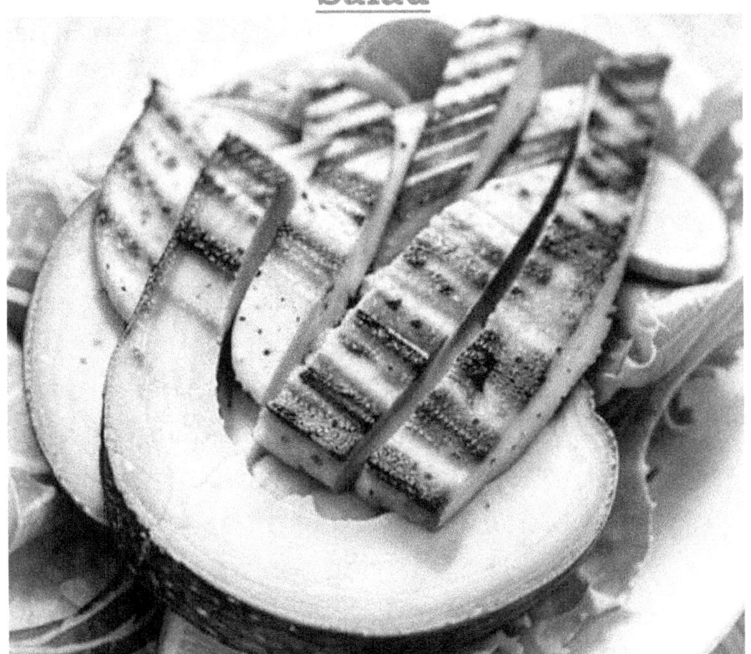

Ingredients:

- Two boneless, skinless chicken breasts
- Two ripe avocados, peeled and dice
- A quarter cup of diced red onion
- Two tablespoons of olive oil
- One lime's juice

- A pinch of salt and pepper, to taste -
  A few fresh cilantro leaves, if desired

Instructions:

- A sizable skillet or grill pan should be preheated in step 1.
- Sprinkle salt and pepper over the chicken breasts after brushing them with olive oil. Cook the chicken for about 8 minutes, or until it is thoroughly cooked, in the heated skillet or grill pan.
- Remove the chicken from the fire and let it to cool for a while.
- Combine diced avocado, red onion, and cilantro (if using) in a big bowl.
- Add the chicken strips that have been cut into strips to the bowl.
- Add salt and pepper to taste and drizzle olive oil and lime juice over the chicken and avocado.
- If desired, serve over a bed of crisp salad leaves. Enjoy!

Vegetable and Lentil Stew

Ingredients:

- 1 chopped onion and 2 tablespoons of olive oil
- 2 minced garlic cloves

- 1 teaspoon smoked paprika - 1 teaspoon dried rosemary
- 3 carrots, chopped - 1/2 tsp. dry thyme
- 1 large, diced russet potato
- 1 cup green lentils, dry
- 2 cups chopped tomatoes - 4 cups vegetable broth
- To taste, add salt and pepper - Optional: add 1/4 cup finely chopped fresh parsley

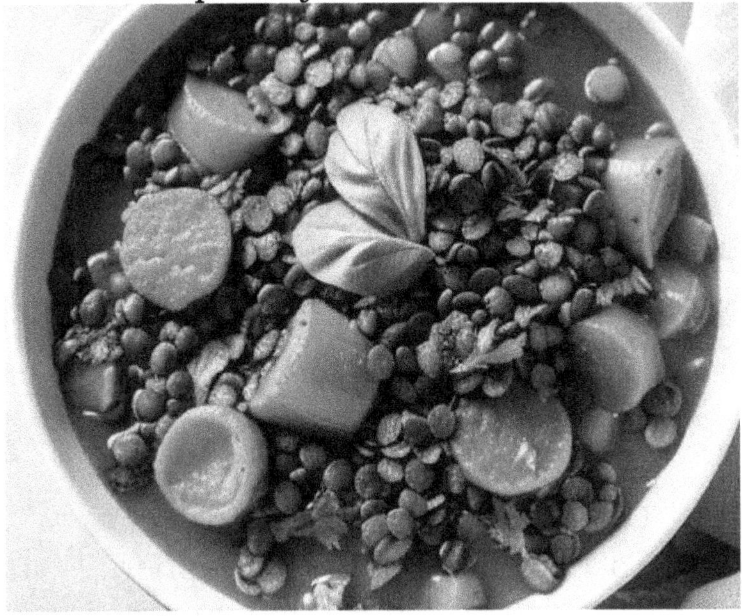

Instructions:

- In a big pot over medium heat, warm the olive oil.

- Add the onion and garlic and simmer for about 5 minutes, or until tender.
- Include the potatoes, carrots, and smoked paprika. Cook for an additional 5 minutes.
- Include the diced tomatoes, vegetable broth, and lentils.
- Bring to a boil, lower the heat, and simmer for approximately 25 minutes, or until the veggies and lentils are soft.
- Salt and pepper should be used to taste.
- If desired, top with chopped parsley and serve hot. Enjoy!

Roasted Veggie Quinoa Bowl

Ingredients:

- 2 cups cooked quinoa; 2 sweet potatoes; 2 diced red bell peppers; 1 cup cooked black beans; and 2 teaspoons olive oil.
- one teaspoon of smoked paprika
- One teaspoon of garlic powder
- To taste, add salt and pepper - You can also add 1/4 cup chopped fresh cilantro.

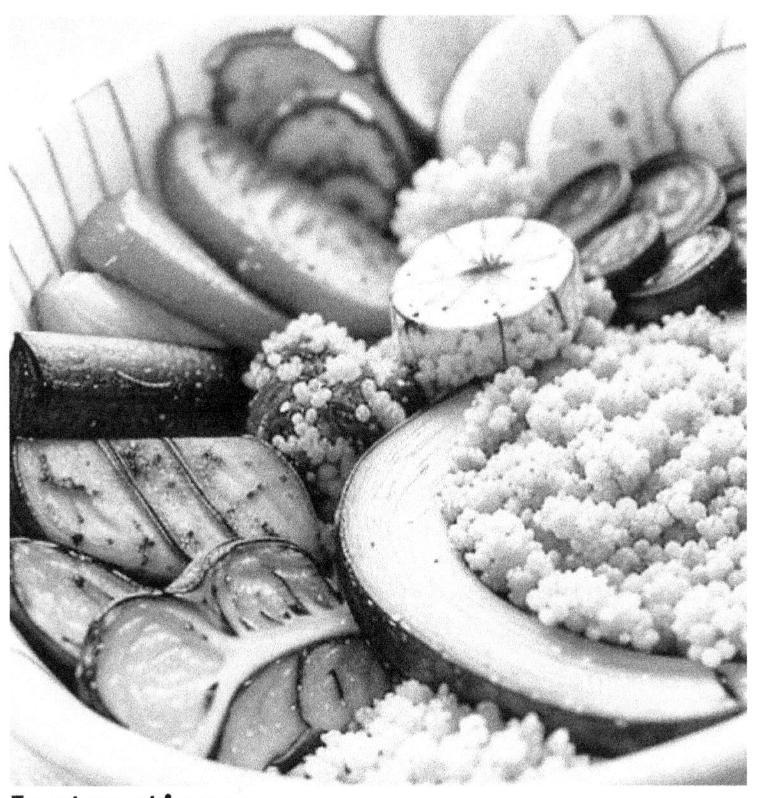

Instructions:

- Start by setting the oven to 375°F (190°C).
- Arrange bell peppers and sweet potatoes on a sizable baking sheet. Drizzle with olive oil.
- Add salt, pepper, smoked paprika, garlic powder, and toss to combine.
- Roast the vegetables for 25 to 30 minutes, or until they are soft.

- Combine cooked quinoa, roasted veggies, and black beans in a big bowl.
- If preferred, top with chopped cilantro and add salt and pepper to suit.
- Present hot. Enjoy!

Eggs with Sweet Potato Hash

Ingredients:
- 2 tablespoons extra virgin olive oil 2 diced sweet potatoes 1 diced red onion 1 diced red bell pepper
- a single teaspoon of smoked paprika
- 1.25 teaspoons of garlic powder
- 4 eggs
- To taste, add salt and pepper
- Optional -- Add a few sprigs of fresh parsley

Instructions:
- In a large skillet, set over medium-high heat, pour in the olive oil and allow it to warm until it is hot enough to sizzle when an ingredient is added.
- Include the bell pepper, onion, and sweet potatoes.

- Boil the potatoes for 10 minutes or until they are soft enough to easily be pierced with a fork or knife.
- Include the garlic powder, smoked paprika, and salt and pepper to taste.
- Crack the eggs into the skillet, leaving space between each one to prevent them from mixing.
- Cook the eggs in the covered skillet until they are done to your preference.
- If wanted, top with freshly chopped parsley and serve warm. Enjoy!

Poached egg with avocado toast

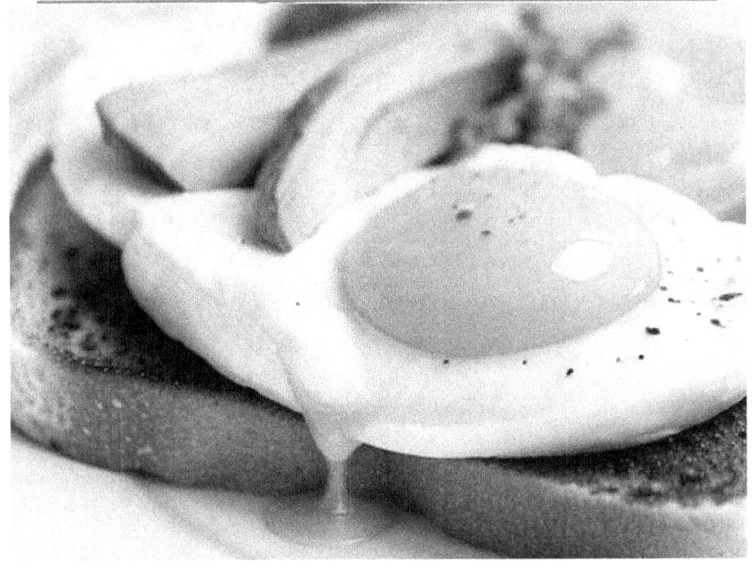

Ingredients:

- 2 slices of your favorite toast,
- 1 ripe avocado, and 2 eggs.
- 2 tablespoons white vinegar,
- 2 peppercorns, and salt to taste
- A few optional fresh cilantro sprigs

Instructions:

- Simmer some water in a small pot.
- Mash the avocado and distribute it on the toast in the meantime.
- Add the vinegar after the water is simmering, then carefully lower the eggs into the water.
- Simmer for 3 to 4 minutes, depending on how done you like your eggs.
- Using a slotted spoon, remove the eggs from the water and put them on the avocado toast.
- If preferred, top with fresh cilantro that has been chopped along with salt and pepper. Enjoy!

CHAPTER 4

Satisfying Dinners
Baked Salmon with Asparagus

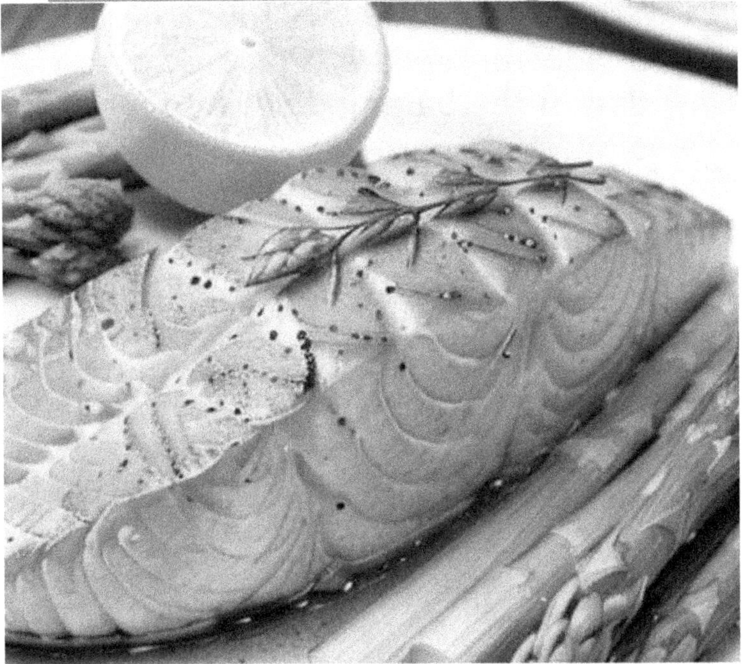

Ingredients:

- 4 fresh salmon fillets (6 ounces each)
- 1 pound of asparagus 4 tablespoons of olive oil
- 2 teaspoons of dried oregano
- 2 minced garlic cloves
- To taste, salt and pepper

Instructions:

- Set the oven to 350 degrees. Salmon fillets should be seasoned with oregano, garlic, salt, and pepper on a baking dish.
- Trim the asparagus's rough ends and divide the spears. Place next to the fish in the baking dish. Add a drizzle of olive oil.
- Bake the salmon and asparagus for 20 minutes, or until the asparagus is tender and the fish is cooked through. Serve.

Turkey and Vegetable Stir-Fry

Ingredients:
- 1Pound lean ground turkey,
- 1 yellow onion, 1 red bell pepper,
- 1 green bell pepper, and 2 minced garlic cloves.
- 2 tablespoons low sodium soy sauce
- 1 tablespoon freshly grated ginger
- 2 tablespoons sesame oil - 2 cups brown rice that has been cooked

Instructions:
- Turn on the medium-high heat under a sizable skillet. Use a spatula or wooden spoon to break up the ground turkey while it cooks until it is no longer pink.
- Stir-fry for 2 minutes after adding the bell peppers, onions, garlic, and ginger.
- Stir-fry for 2 more minutes after adding the soy sauce and sesame oil.
- Stir-fry the cooked rice for one minute after adding it. Stir-fry is best served hot.

Cauliflower Rice Pilaf

Ingredients:
- 1 grated head of cauliflower
- 2 tablespoons of extra virgin olive oil

- 1 diced onion - 1 diced carrot
- 1 diced red bell pepper
- 3 minced garlic cloves
- Paprika, 1 teaspoon
- 1/4 cup freshly grated Parmesan cheese
- 2 tablespoons finely chopped fresh parsley - Salt and pepper to taste

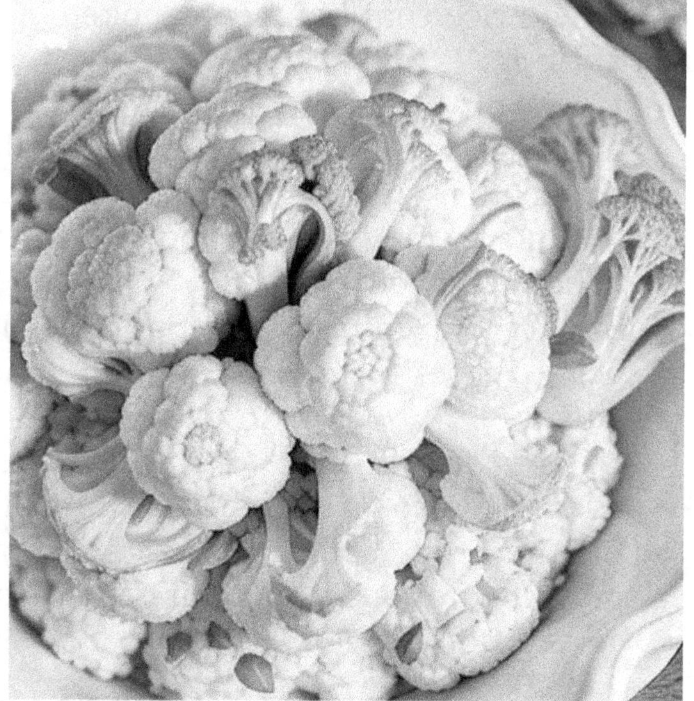

Instructions:

- In a large skillet on a medium-high heat, gradually warm the olive oil.

- Add the bell pepper, bell pepper, onions, and garlic and sauté for about 5 minutes, or until the vegetables are tender.
- Include the grated cauliflower and season to taste with salt, pepper, paprika, and parsley. Cook the cauliflower for a further 8 to 10 minutes, or until it is soft.
- After taking it off the heat, whisk in the Parmesan cheese. Serve warm.

Oatmeal Banana Pancakes

Ingredients:

- 1 cup rolled oats
- 1 mashed ripe banana
- 1/4 cup Greek yogurt, plain
- A quantity of approximately one half of a teaspoon of baking powder is required.
- 1/4 teaspoon cinnamon, ground
- 2 eggs
- milk, 2 tablespoons
- 1 teaspoon of honey

Instructions:

- With a fork, mash the banana in a bowl until it is completely smooth.
- Include the oats, Greek yogurt, baking soda, cinnamon, eggs, milk, and honey. Whisk everything together until the mixture is smooth and all the ingredients are mixed.
- Spray cooking spray into a non-stick skillet and preheat it over medium heat.
- Using a 1/4 cup measuring cup, pour the batter onto the hot skillet and cook for 1–2 minutes, or until the edges begin to become golden brown. When the pancake is cooked

through, flip it over and cook for an additional 1-2 minutes.
- Continue using the remaining batter. Serve with honey or slices of fresh banana.

Zucchini and Feta Frittata

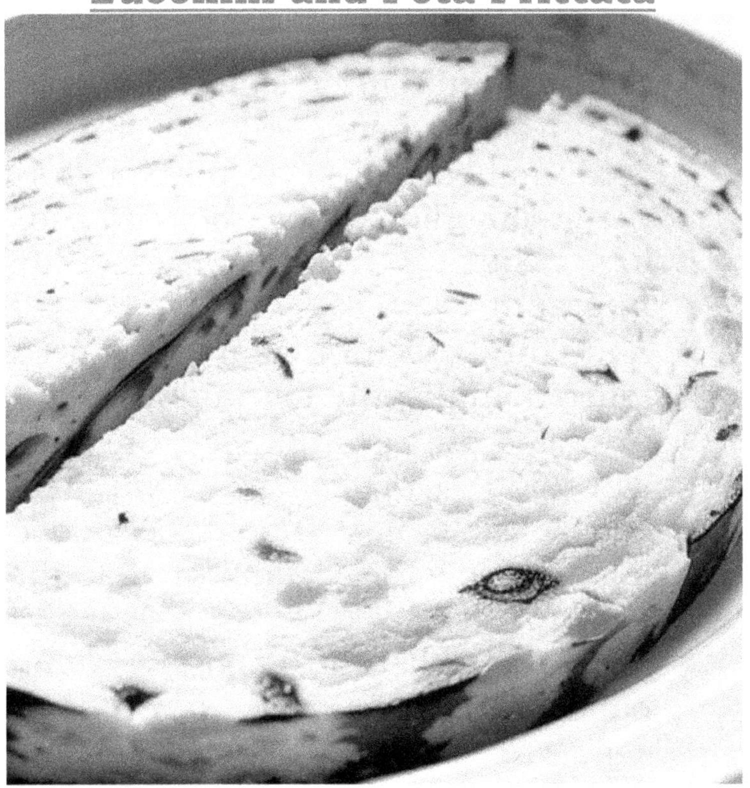

Ingredients:
- 1 sliced green onion and
- 1 tablespoon of olive oil
- 2 minced garlic cloves

- 1 minced big zucchini
- 4 lightly beaten eggs
- 2 teaspoons of recently cut parsley
- 1 tsp. dried oregano
- A dash of salt and pepper - 1/4 cup feta cheese crumbles

Instructions:

- Set the oven to 375 degrees.
- In an oven-safe skillet set over medium heat, warm the olive oil. Add the green onion and garlic, and cook for about 2 minutes, or until fragrant.
- Add the zucchini that has been minced, and sauté for 5 minutes.
- Combine the eggs, parsley, oregano, salt, and pepper in a bowl. Feta cheese crumbles should be added after pouring the egg mixture into the skillet.
- Place the skillet in the hot oven, and bake for 15-20 minutes, or until the eggs are set and just beginning to turn brown. Serve hot.

CHAPTER 5

Vegetarian PCOS-Friendly recipes

Spinach and Chickpea Power Salad

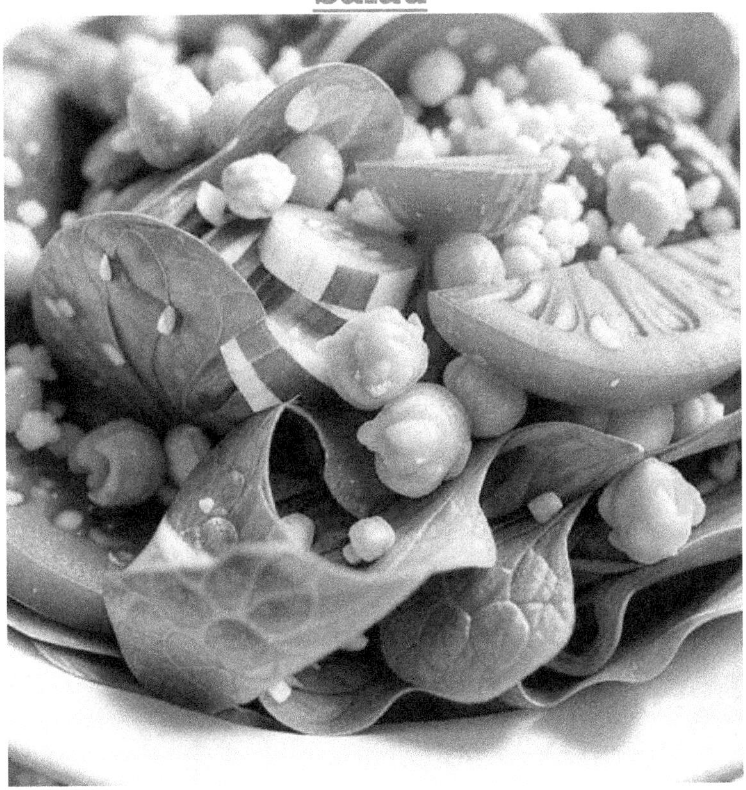

Ingredients:

- 5 cups chopped spinach
- 1 can washed and drained chickpeas

- 1/2 cup chopped roasted red peppers
- 1/2 cup crumbled feta cheese
- 1/2 teaspoon garlic powder,
- 1/4 cup pepitas (pumpkin seeds),
- 2 teaspoons red wine vinegar, and
- 2 tablespoons olive oil.
- One-half teaspoon oregano
- To taste, salt and pepper

Instructions:

- Combine the spinach, chickpeas, feta cheese, pepitas, and roasted red peppers in a big bowl.
- Combine the red wine vinegar, olive oil, oregano, garlic powder, salt, and pepper in a separate small bowl.
- Pour the salad with the dressing, then toss to incorporate.
- Dish out and savour!

Cauliflower Rice Stir-Fry with Tofu

Ingredients:

- 2 tablespoons sesame oil, 1/2 cup sliced onion, and
- 1 tablespoon minced garlic
- 1 chopped red bell pepper
- 1/2 pound of cubed firm tofu

- 1 cup frozen peas - 2 tablespoons soy sauce - 2 cups cauliflower rice
- One tablespoon Sriracha
- To taste, salt and pepper

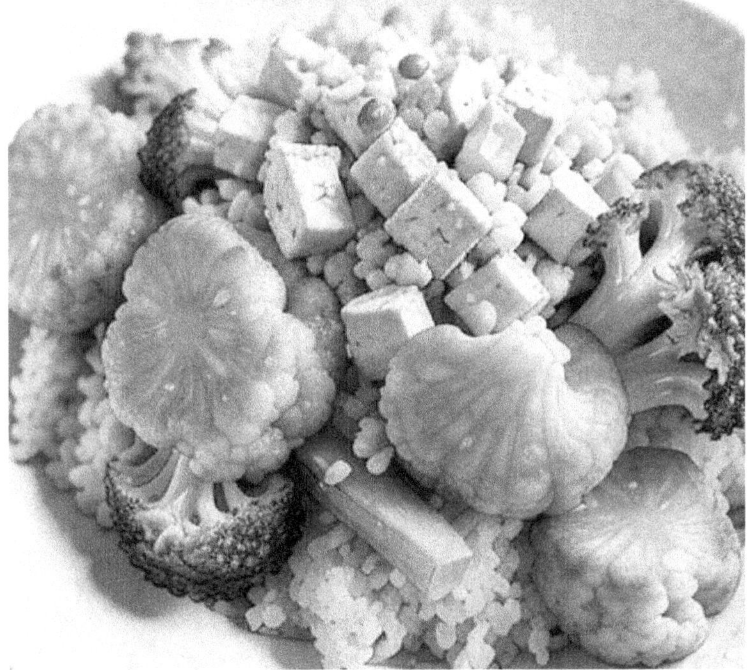

Instructions:

- In a large skillet over medium heat, warm the sesame oil.
- Include the onion, garlic, and bell pepper and sauté for 5 minutes or until the vegetables are tender.

- Include the tofu and cook for a further 5 minutes, or until golden brown.
- Add the soy sauce, sriracha, cauliflower rice, peas, and mix to incorporate.
- Cook for about 10 minutes, stirring periodically, or until the cauliflower is soft.
- To taste, add salt and pepper.
- Plate and savour!

Lentil and Vegetable Curry Delight

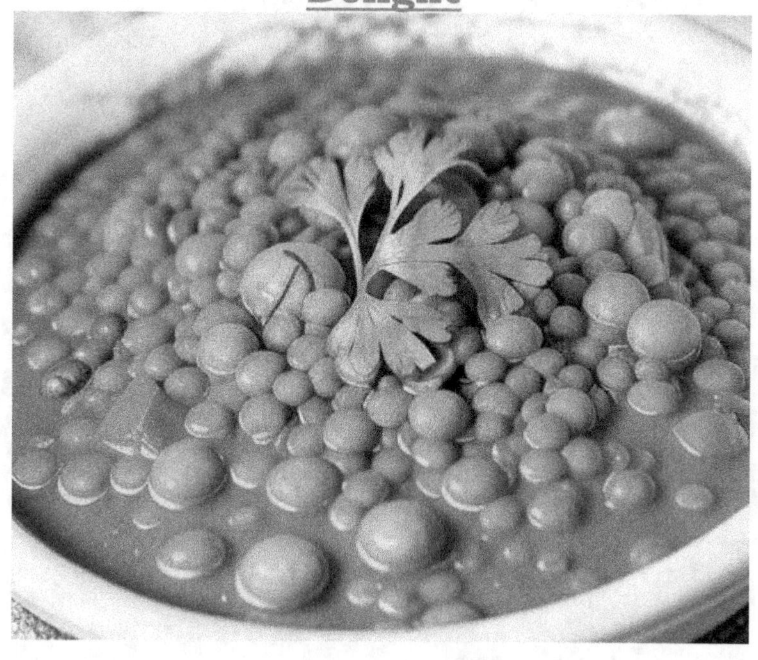

Ingredients:

- 2 minced garlic cloves
- 1/2 cup chopped onion
- 1 tablespoon of olive oil
- Curry powder, two tablespoons
- One-half of a teaspoon of ground coriander and one teaspoon of cumin.
- One-fourth teaspoon turmeric
- 1/2 cup carrots, chopped
- 1 chopped red bell pepper
- 1 can (15 ounces) washed and drained lentils
- One 15-ounce can of diced tomatoes
- Half a cup of coconut milk
- To taste, salt and pepper

Instructions:

- In a large pot placed over medium heat, pour in the olive oil and allow it to heat until it is comfortably warmed.
- Add the onion and garlic and sauté for about 5 minutes, or until tender.
- Stir the curry powder, cumin, coriander, and turmeric for about a minute or until aromatic.

- Add the bell pepper and carrots, and sauté for about 5 minutes, stirring regularly, until softened.
- Include the coconut milk, tomatoes, and lentils and whisk everything together.
- Bring the mixture to a boil, lower the heat, and simmer for 15 minutes while stirring regularly.
- To taste, add salt and pepper to the dish.
- Dish out and savour!

Zucchini Noodles with Creamy Avocado Sauce

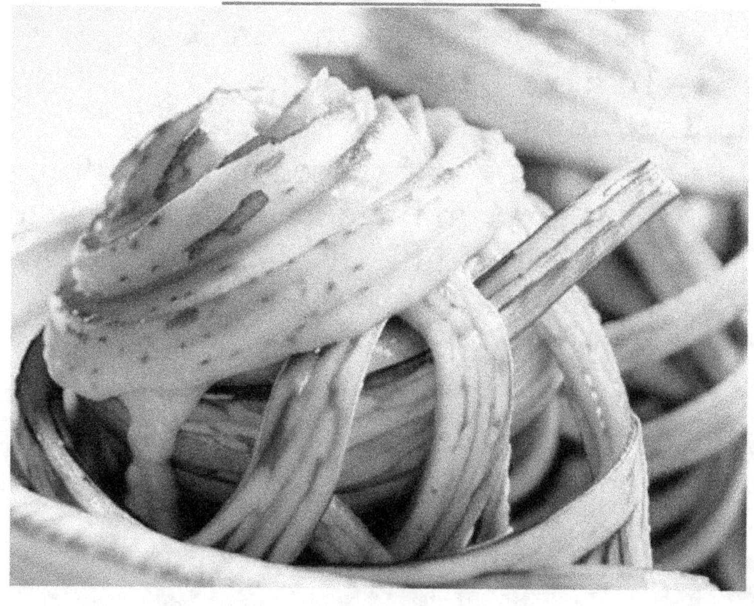

Ingredients:
- 2 spiralized zucchini,
- 2 tablespoons olive oil,
- 1/2 cup diced onion, 1 pitted and peeled avocado,
- 1/4 cup chopped fresh cilantro, and 1/4 cup plain Greek yogurt.
- 1-teaspoon lime juice
- 1/4 teaspoon dried garlic
- To taste, salt and pepper

Instructions:
- In a large skillet heated over medium heat, pour in the olive oil and allow it to warm.
- Include the onion and simmer for about 5 minutes, or until tender.
- Add the zucchini noodles and simmer for about 5 minutes, stirring periodically, until tender.
- Combine the avocado, cilantro, Greek yogurt, lime juice, garlic powder, salt, and pepper in a blender or food processor.
- Process ingredients in a blender until they are combined and form a sauce that is smooth in consistency.

- Cover the zucchini noodles with the sauce and toss to mix.
- Plate and savour!

Quinoa Stuffed Bell Peppers

Ingredients:

- 4 bell peppers, tops removed and seeds removed;
- 1 tablespoon extra-virgin olive oil; 1/2 cup diced onion;
- 1 teaspoon minced garlic.
- 1 serving of cooked quinoa
- 1 can of black beans (15 ounces), drained and rinsed
- 1 can of corn (15 ounces)
- 1/4 cup chopped fresh cilantro
- 1/2 cup enchilada sauce.
- 1 cup of cheddar cheese, shredded

Instructions:

- Dry off the bell peppers and preheat the oven to 375°F.
- In a big skillet over medium heat, warm the olive oil.
- Add the onion and garlic, and cook for about 5 minutes, or until tender.
- Stir in the enchilada sauce, quinoa, black beans, corn, and cilantro.

- Fill the bell peppers as much as possible by dividing the mixture among them.
- Put the bell peppers in a baking dish and cover them with the enchilada sauce.
- Sprinkle some cheddar cheese shredded over each bell pepper.
- Bake for about 15 minutes, or until the cheese is melted and bubbling.
- Plate and savour!

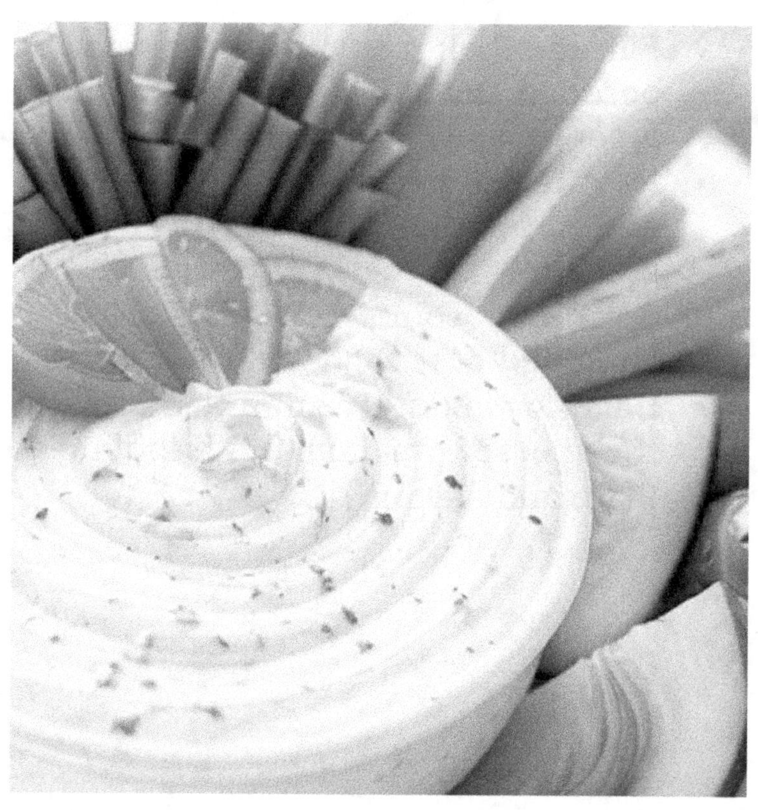

CHAPTER 6

Snacks with a Purpose
Crunchy Chickpea Snack

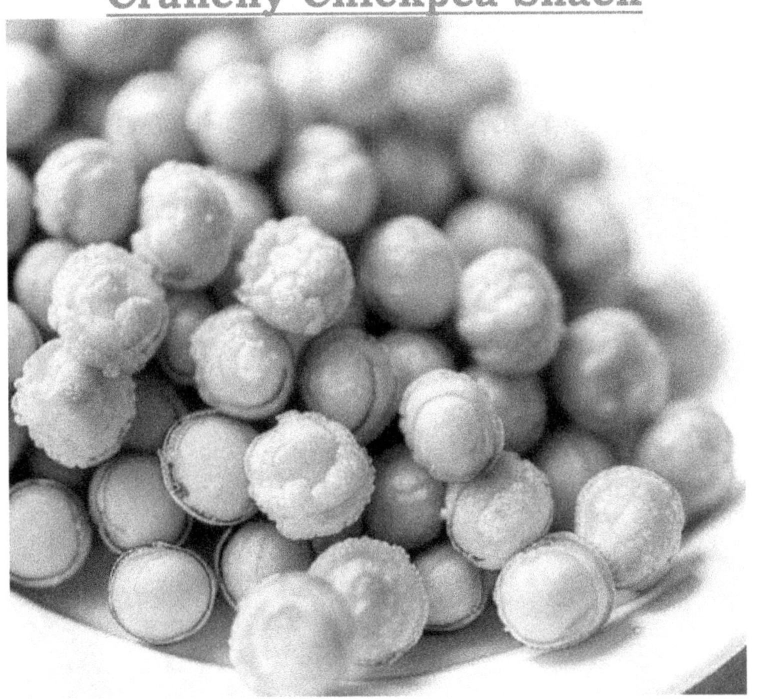

Ingredients:

- 1 can washed and drained chickpeas; 2 tablespoons olive oil; 1 teaspoon garlic powder.
- A half teaspoon of paprika
- One-half teaspoon cumin
- To taste, salt and pepper

Instructions:

- Set oven temperature to 400°F (200°C).
- Scatter the washed, drained chickpeas over a parchment-lined baking sheet.
- Drizzle with olive oil and season with salt, pepper, cumin, paprika, and garlic powder.
- Bake chickpeas for 25 to 30 minutes, or until they are crisp and golden.

Greek Yogurt Dip with Fresh Veggies

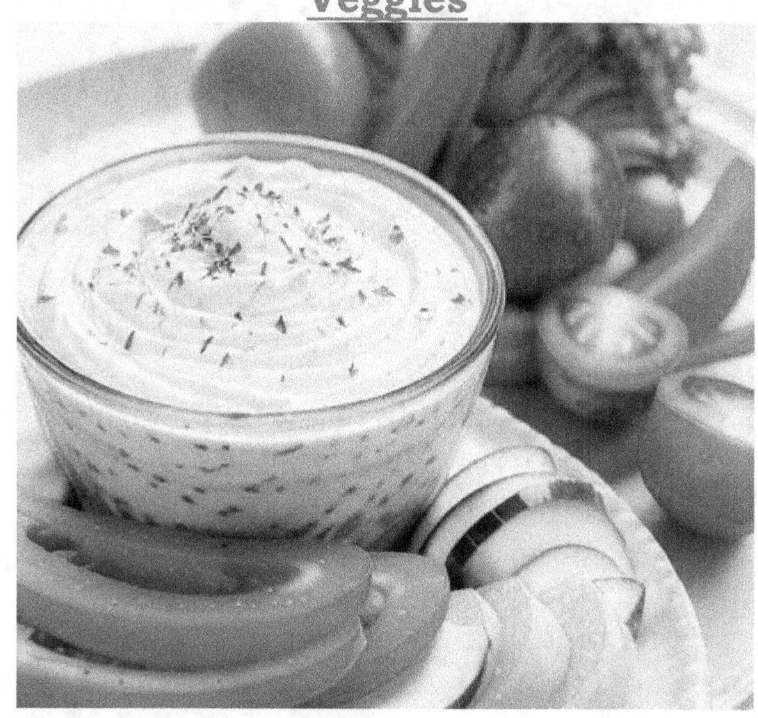

Ingredients:

- 2 cups Greek yogurt that is plain.
- One teaspoon of garlic powder
- 2 tablespoons of dill, 1/2 teaspoon of salt, 1/4 teaspoon of pepper,
- 1 sliced cucumber, and 1 diced red pepper
- 2 grated carrots

Instructions:

- Combine the Greek yogurt, garlic powder, dill, salt, and pepper in a medium bowl.
- Stir the dip ingredients together after adding the diced cucumber, red pepper, and grated carrot.
- Provide crackers or raw vegetables for dipping.

Almonds and Berries Mix

Ingredients:

- 1/2 cup dried cranberries and
- 1 cup almonds.
- 1/2 cup blueberries, dried
- A half-cup of dried cherries

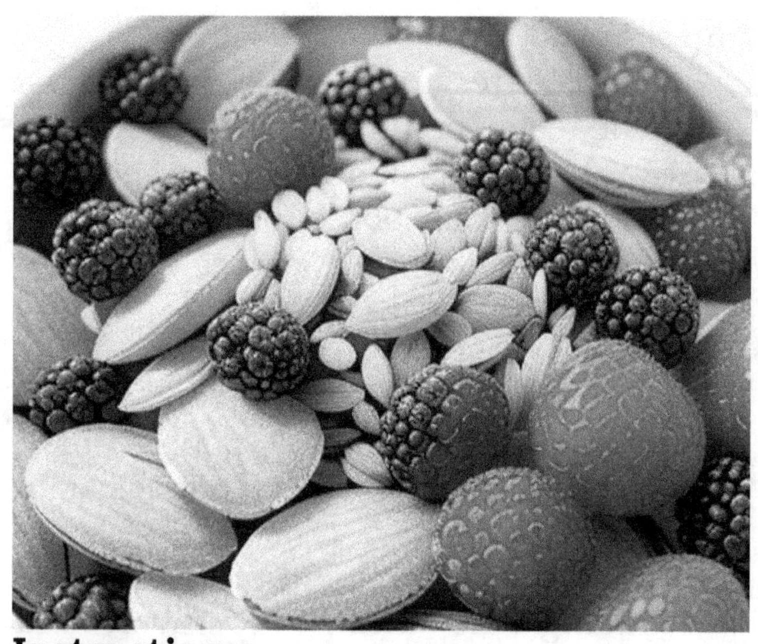

Instructions:

- Set oven temperature to 350°F (180°C).
- Spread the almonds out on a baking sheet and roast for 7 to 10 minutes, or until golden brown.
- Take the food out of the oven and let it cool.
- Combine the toasted almonds, dried cranberries, dried blueberries, and dried cherries in a medium bowl.
- Ensure that the item is placed in a tightly sealed container before storing it in the refrigerator.

CHAPTER 7

Power-Packed Smoothies
Green Goddess Smoothie

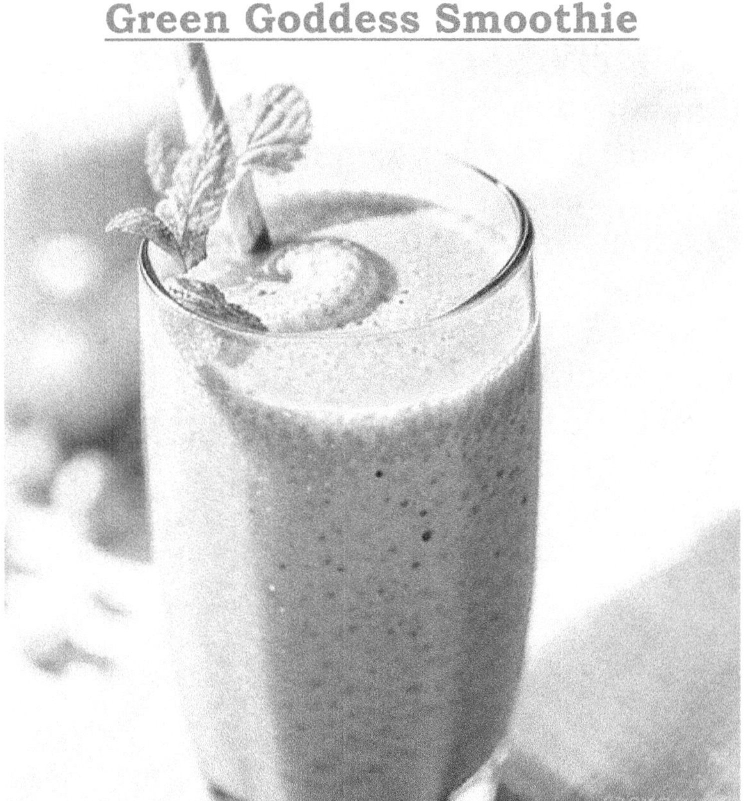

Ingredients:
- a large, ripe banana that has been peeled and chopped into bits; one cup of fresh spinach;
- half a cup of unsweetened almond milk; one tablespoon of honey; and

one-half teaspoon of ground cinnamon.

- 1/4 teaspoon each of ground ginger and ground nutmeg
- Half a cup of Greek yogurt

Instructions:

- In a blender, combine the spinach, banana, almond milk, honey, cinnamon, ginger, and nutmeg. Until smooth, blend.
- Add the yogurt and mix well to incorporate.
- Divide the smoothie between two cups and serve.

Berry Blast Protein Shake

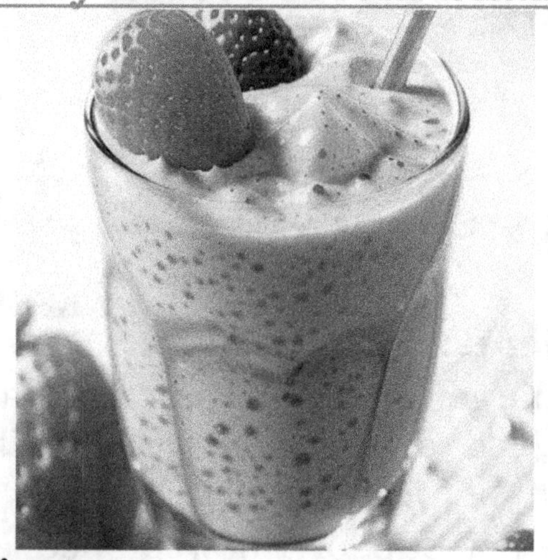

Ingredients:

- 1 cup frozen mixed berries

- 1/2 cup plain Greek yogurt.
- 1 scoop whey protein powder
- 1/2 cup almond milk
- One teaspoon of honey

Instructions:

- Combine all ingredients in a blender, and process for 30 seconds, or until completely smooth.
- Divide the mixture among two glasses in order to provide a serving of the mixture for each person.

Chocolate Banana Smoothie

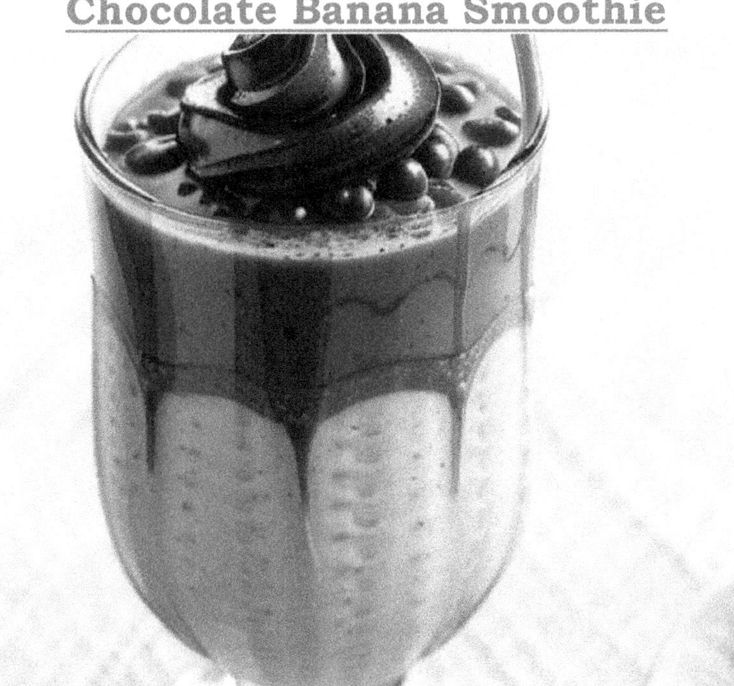

Ingredients:

- 2 ripe bananas, peeled and sliced into pieces.
- One cup of almond milk
- cocoa powder, 2 teaspoons
- One-half teaspoon of cinnamon combined with one tablespoon of honey.

Instructions:
- In a blender, combine the bananas, almond milk, chocolate powder, honey, and cinnamon.
- Purée until fluid.
- Fill two glasses with the liquid and serve.

CHAPTER 8

Delicious Desserts

Mixed-berry Chia Seed Pudding

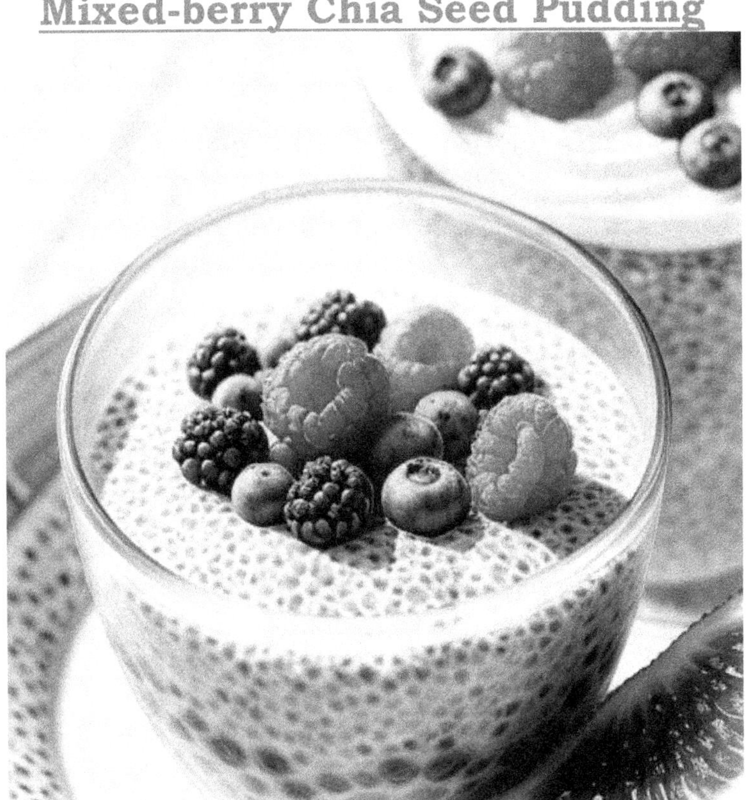

Ingredients:

- 1/4 cup chia seeds - 2 cups almond milk
- 2 cups of mixed berries and 2 tablespoons of honey

Instructions:

- Combine the almond milk, chia seeds, and honey in a medium bowl.
- Combine everything thoroughly by mixing.
- Place the bowl in the refrigerator to chill for at least two hours, then cover with a lid or plastic wrap.
- Once the chia pudding has cooled, give it a couple stirs to make it creamy.
- Distribute the pudding into four small bowls or glasses.
- Add the berries on top.
- Plate and savour!

Baked Apples with Cinnamon

Ingredients:
- 4 cored apples, 2 tablespoons melted butter,
- 2 tablespoons honey, and 1 teaspoon cinnamon.
- 2 Tbsp raisins (optional)
- 1 Tbsp coconut sugar

Instructions:
- Set oven to 350 degrees Fahrenheit.
- Put the apple cores in a baking tray.

- Combine the melted butter, honey, cinnamon, and coconut sugar in a small bowl.
- After adding the apples, gently stir the mixture.
- Put the prepared dish in the oven and bake for 30 minutes.
- If using, add the raisins and bake a further 15 minutes.
- Plate warm, and savor!

Dark Chocolate Avocado Mousse

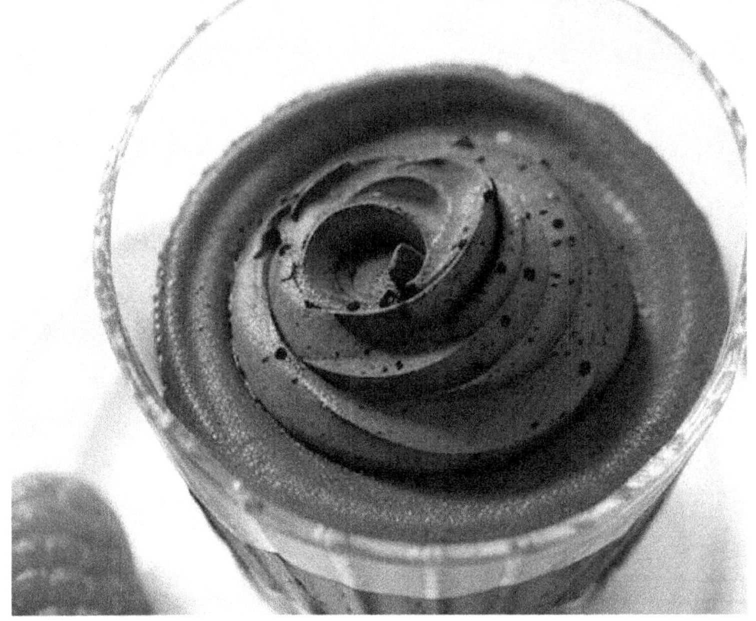

Ingredients:

- two ripe avocados and one-fourth cup of cocoa powder.
- 2 tablespoons of honey
- 1/4 cup melted dark chocolate
- One-fourth cup almond milk
- Optional garnishes include whipped cream, berries, and chopped nuts.

Instructions:

- Combine the avocados, cocoa powder, honey, and dark chocolate in a blender or food processor and mix until smooth.
- When necessary to achieve desired consistency, add almond milk.
- Distribute the mousse among four small cups or bowls.
- Optional toppings include whipped cream, berries, or chopped almonds.
- Present and savour!

CHAPTER 9

Herbal Teas for PCOS Management

1. Minty Hormone Harmony Tea

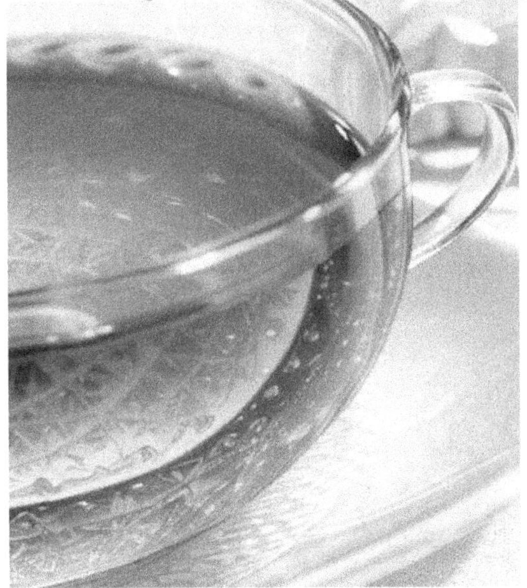

An energizing, minty tea combination called Harmony Tea supports hormonal balance.

2. Cinnamon Spice Infusion

To balance hormone levels, this warm and spiciness blend of cinnamon, cardamom, ginger, and cloves.

3. Lavender and Chamomile Relaxation Blend

This blend of chamomile and lavender is calming and relaxing, lowering stress levels and supporting the endocrine system.

4. Fenugreek and Fennel Supportive Tea

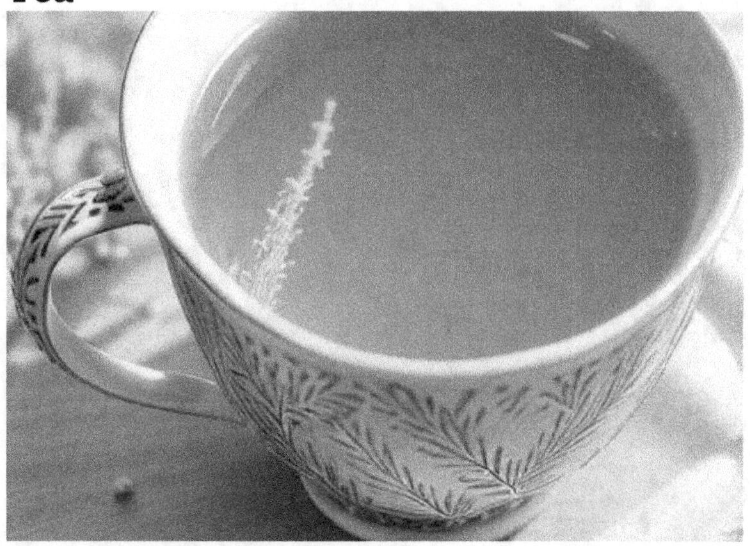

An endocrine system-supporting mix of fenugreek and fennel.

5. Spearmint and Licorice Root Balance Brew

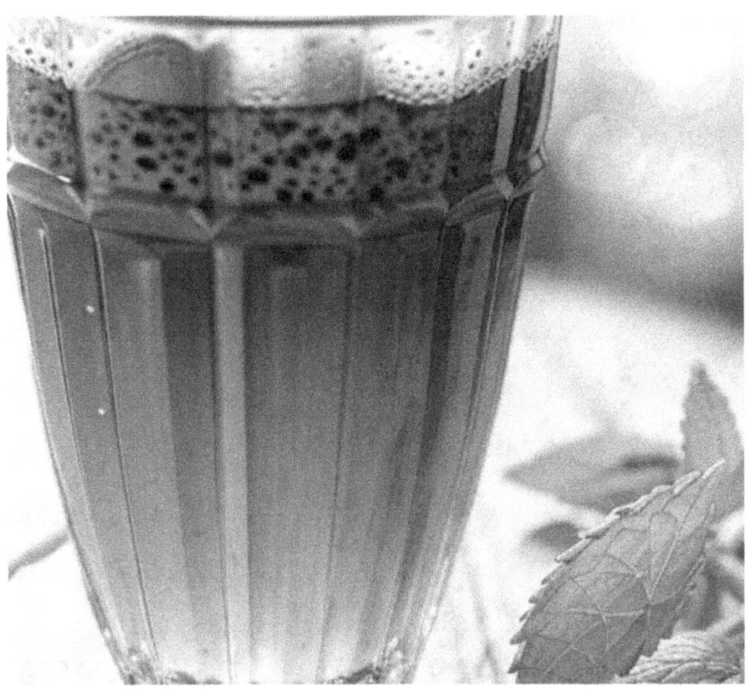

This tea combines licorice root and spearmint to help regulate hormones.

6. Nettle Leaf Nourishing Infusion

This infusion of nettle leaves is nutritious and supports hormone control.

7. Raspberry Leaf Reproductive Wellness Tea

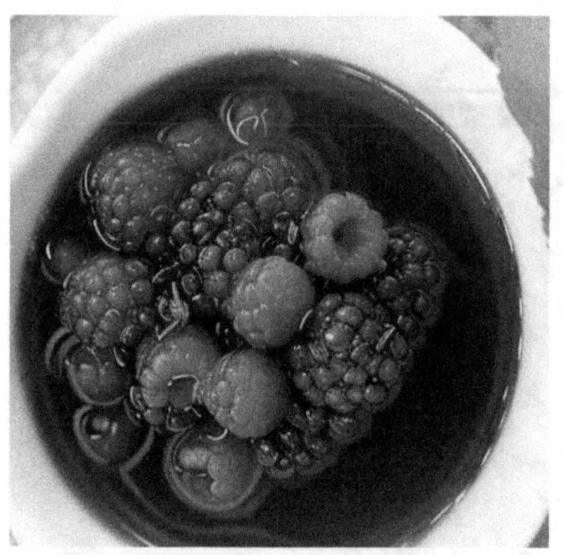

A light raspberry leaf blend to promote general reproductive health.

8. Ginger Turmeric Anti-Inflammatory Elixir

A hot concoction of ginger and turmeric that helps the endocrine system and reduces inflammation.

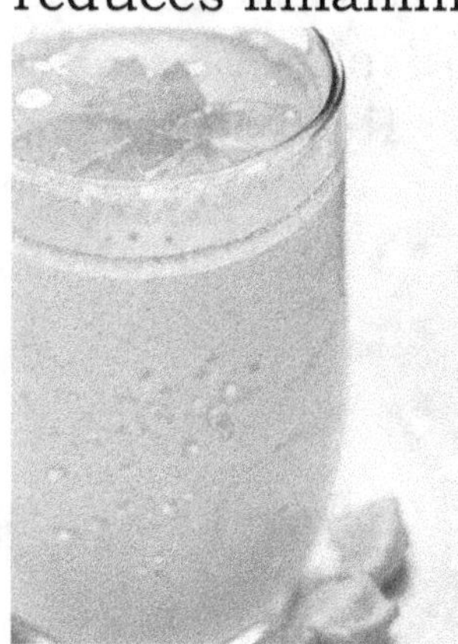

CHAPTER 10

7-Day Meal Plan

DAY 1

Breakfast	Lunch	Dinner
Vegetable Omelette	Eggs with Sweet Potato Hash	Cauliflower Rice Pilaf

DAY 2

Breakfast	Lunch	Dinner
Spinach and Mushroom Breakfast Wrap	Poached egg with avocado toast	Zucchini and Feta Frittata

DAY 3

Breakfast	Lunch	Dinner
Berry and Greek Yogurt Parfait	Roasted Veggie Quinoa Bowl	Turkey and Vegetable Stir-Fry

DAY 4

Breakfast	Lunch	Dinner
Berry and Greek Yogurt Parfait	Avocado with Grilled Chicken Salad	Oatmeal Banana Pancakes

DAY 5

Breakfast	Lunch	Dinner
Spinach and Mushroom Breakfast Wrap	Vegetable and Lentil Stew	Baked Salmon with Asparagus

DAY 6

Breakfast	Lunch	Dinner
Veggie-Packed Breakfast Burritos	Eggs with Sweet Potato Hash	Oatmeal Banana Pancakes

DAY 7

Breakfast	Lunch	Dinner
Vegetable Omelette	Roasted Veggie Quinoa Bowl	Turkey and Vegetable Stir-Fry

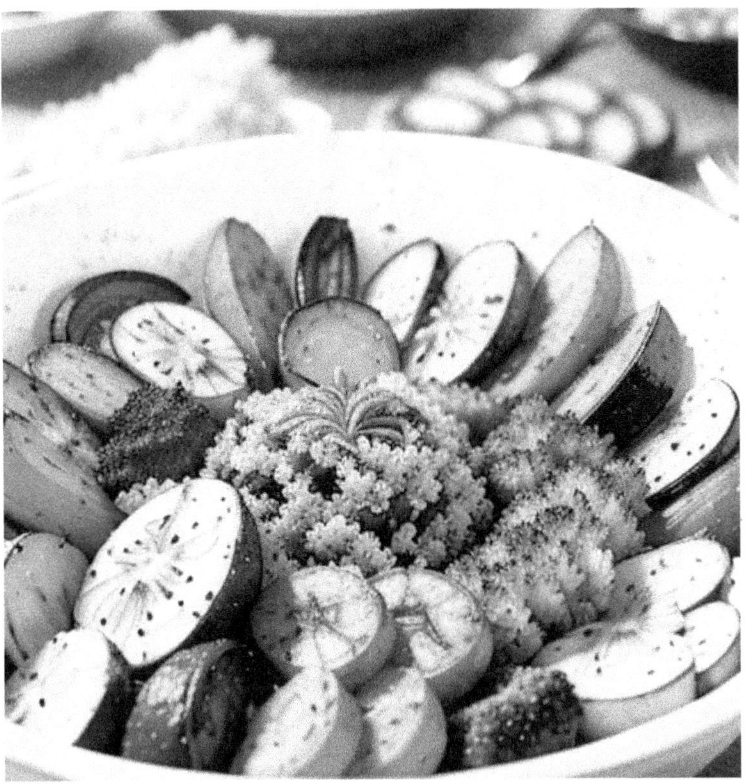

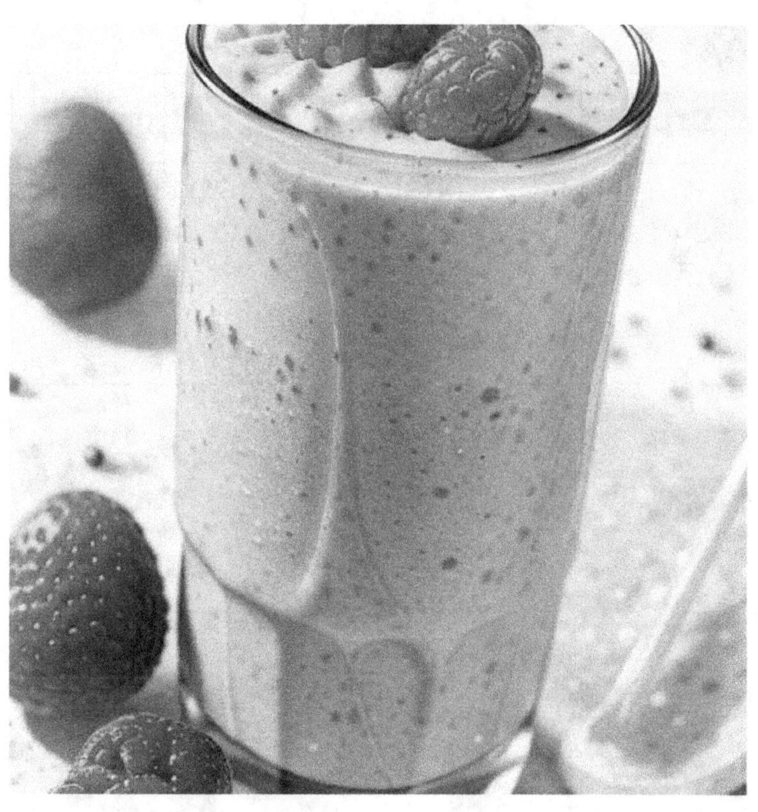

CONCLUSION

This PCOS Recipes Cookbook for Beginners is a life-changing resource for anyone looking to manage PCOS through tasty, conscious eating. This cookbook gives novices the tools they need to take control of their health and wellbeing by offering a wide variety of dishes designed specifically for the special requirements of people with PCOS.

This cookbook's pages have examined the artistry of preparing wholesome, well-balanced meals that not only help hormone management but also indulge the senses. We have embraced the idea that eating healthfully can be pleasant and fun by emphasizing whole, nutrient-dense foods and adding a range of flavours and textures.

The recipes in these pages are intended to promote progress rather than perfection because changing one's diet can be a gradual process. Every step you take to develop healthy habits is a victory, and this cookbook is here to help you along the way.

Take the time to taste the flavours as you So may this cookbook be your dependable travel companion as you pursue a balanced and PCOS-friendly way of life, whether you're whipping up a quick and simple breakfast, cooking a hearty supper, or indulging in a guilt-free dessert. Let's enjoy the benefits of mindful eating, embrace the joy of cooking, and eventually thrive despite PCOS.

I'm grateful that you took the time to read my book. I hope you like it and it gave you something to think about. Thank You

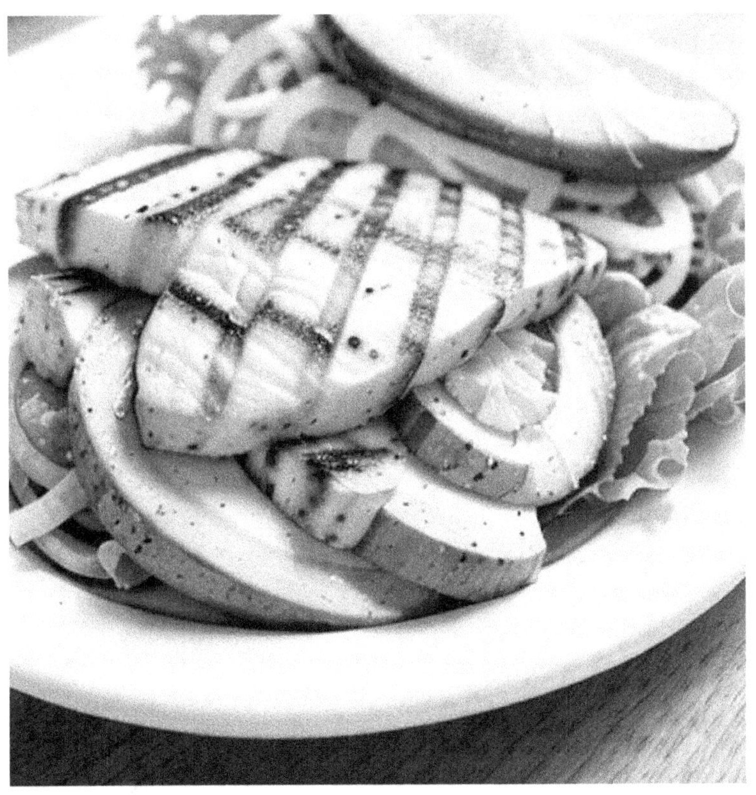

Weekly Meal Planner

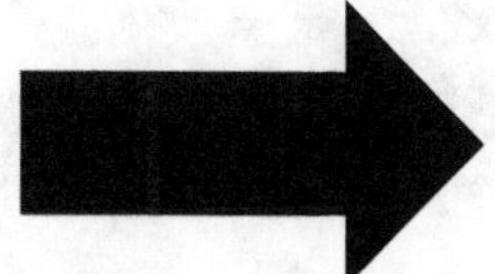

MONDAY	B	
	L	
	D	
TUESDAY	B	
	L	
	D	
WENESDAY	B	
	L	
	D	
THURSDAY	B	
	L	
	D	
FRIDAY	B	
	L	
	D	
SATURDAY	B	
	L	
	D	
SUNDAY	B	
	L	
	D	

MONDAY	B	
	L	
	D	
TUESDAY	B	
	L	
	D	
WENESDAY	B	
	L	
	D	
THURSDAY	B	
	L	
	D	
FRIDAY	B	
	L	
	D	
SATURDAY	B	
	L	
	D	
SUNDAY	B	
	L	
	D	

MONDAY	B
	L
	D
TUESDAY	B
	L
	D
WENESDAY	B
	L
	D
THURSDAY	B
	L
	D
FRIDAY	B
	L
	D
SATURDAY	B
	L
	D
SUNDAY	B
	L
	D

MONDAY	B
	L
	D

TUESDAY	B
	L
	D

WENESDAY	B
	L
	D

THURSDAY	B
	L
	D

FRIDAY	B
	L
	D

SATURDAY	B
	L
	D

SUNDAY	B
	L
	D

MONDAY	B	
	L	
	D	

TUESDAY	B	
	L	
	D	

WENESDAY	B	
	L	
	D	

THURSDAY	B	
	L	
	D	

FRIDAY	B	
	L	
	D	

SATURDAY	B	
	L	
	D	

SUNDAY	B	
	L	
	D	

MONDAY	B	
	L	
	D	
TUESDAY	**B**	
	L	
	D	
WENESDAY	**B**	
	L	
	D	
THURSDAY	**B**	
	L	
	D	
FRIDAY	**B**	
	L	
	D	
SATURDAY	**B**	
	L	
	D	
SUNDAY	**B**	
	L	
	D	

MONDAY	B	
	L	
	D	
TUESDAY	B	
	L	
	D	
WENESDAY	B	
	L	
	D	
THURSDAY	B	
	L	
	D	
FRIDAY	B	
	L	
	D	
SATURDAY	B	
	L	
	D	
SUNDAY	B	
	L	
	D	

DAILY MEAL PLANNER

TO DO

1	
2	
3	
4	
5	
6	
7	
8	
9	
10	

EXERCISE

GOAL ACTIVITIES

- [ ]
- [ ]
- [ ]
- [ ]
- [ ]
- [ ]
- [ ]

SHOPPING

MEALS	
BREAKFAST	
LUNCH	
DINNER	
SNACKS	
DESSERTS	

OBSERVATION

INSPIRATION

NOTES & TIPS

DAILY MEAL PLANNER

TO DO	
1	
2	
3	
4	
5	
6	
7	
8	
9	
10	

EXERCISE

GOAL ACTIVITIES

	☐
	☐
	☐
	☐
	☐
	☐
	☐

SHOPPING

<table>
<tr><td colspan="2">MEALS</td><td>OBSERVATION</td></tr>
<tr><td>BREAKFAST</td><td></td><td></td></tr>
<tr><td>LUNCH</td><td></td><td></td></tr>
<tr><td>DINNER</td><td></td><td></td></tr>
<tr><td>SNACKS</td><td></td><td>INSPIRATION</td></tr>
<tr><td>DESSERTS</td><td></td><td></td></tr>
</table>

NOTES & TIPS

DAILY MEAL PLANNER

TO DO	
1	
2	
3	
4	
5	
6	
7	
8	
9	
10	

EXERCISE

GOAL ACTIVITIES

- ☐
- ☐
- ☐
- ☐
- ☐
- ☐
- ☐

SHOPPING

<table>
<tr><td colspan="2">MEALS</td><td>OBSERVATION</td></tr>
<tr><td>BREAKFAST</td><td></td><td></td></tr>
<tr><td>LUNCH</td><td></td><td></td></tr>
<tr><td>DINNER</td><td></td><td></td></tr>
<tr><td>SNACKS</td><td></td><td>INSPIRATION</td></tr>
<tr><td>DESSERTS</td><td></td><td></td></tr>
</table>

NOTES & TIPS

www.ingramcontent.com/pod-product-compliance
Lightning Source LLC
Chambersburg PA
CBHW050839260726
48660CB00006B/2335